MY MOMMY HAD BREAST CANCER

By Jaime Alfaro

With Senna Alfaro

For Senna and Tazio,

Thank you for your love and support through my battle with breast cancer. You are amazing kids. You gave and continue to give me strength, hope, and motivation.

This book offers the briefest glimpse into my family's life during my battle with breast cancer through the perspective of my oldest child. My daughter, Senna, was only six-years-old when I was diagnosed. She was so innocent and yet so aware. I wrote this book because I wish that she would have had something like this to prepare her for what was to come when I was diagnosed, as well as to know that she was not alone as a child with a parent battling cancer. My son, Tazio, was also deeply impacted by this battle and was a superstar of a toddler through the whole ordeal. Being newly three when I was diagnosed his experience was vastly different. However, I believe a book like this would have helped him too.

The images in this book are actual snapshots of my family and me throughout our journey from diagnosis through treatment, altered to look like sketches. They are not the typical illustrations you would see in a children's book. These images are intended to help kids see the truth of cancer treatment in a gentle and accessible manner.

If you are reading this book it likely means that you and those you love are impacted by cancer. Please know that you are not alone. Stay strong and fight the good fight.

—JAIME ALFARO

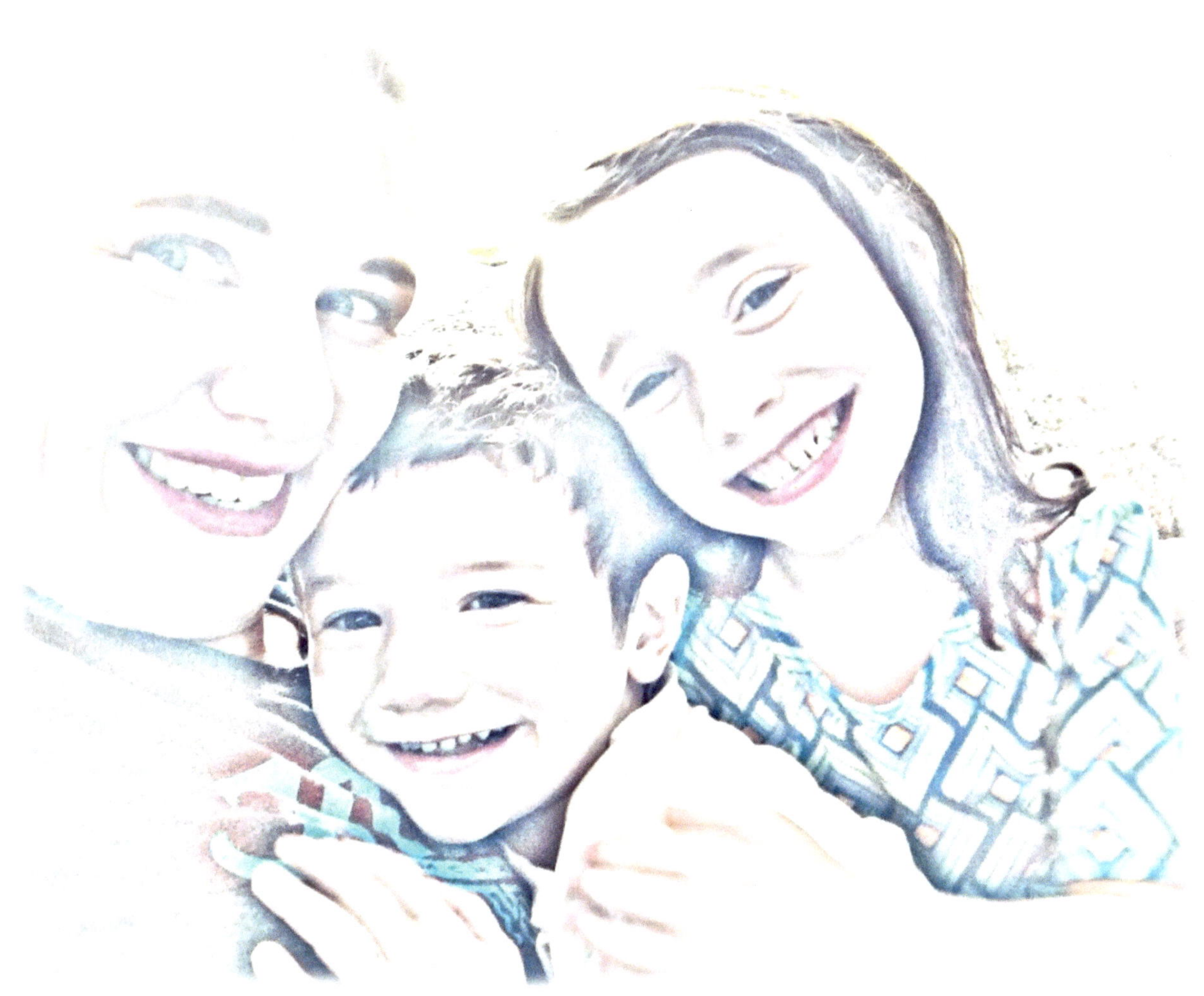

One day Mommy told me that she was sick with something called Breast Cancer. I didn't understand. Mommy seemed fine. She and my little brother had even walked me to school that day. How was she sick? She wasn't coughing and she didn't have a fever.

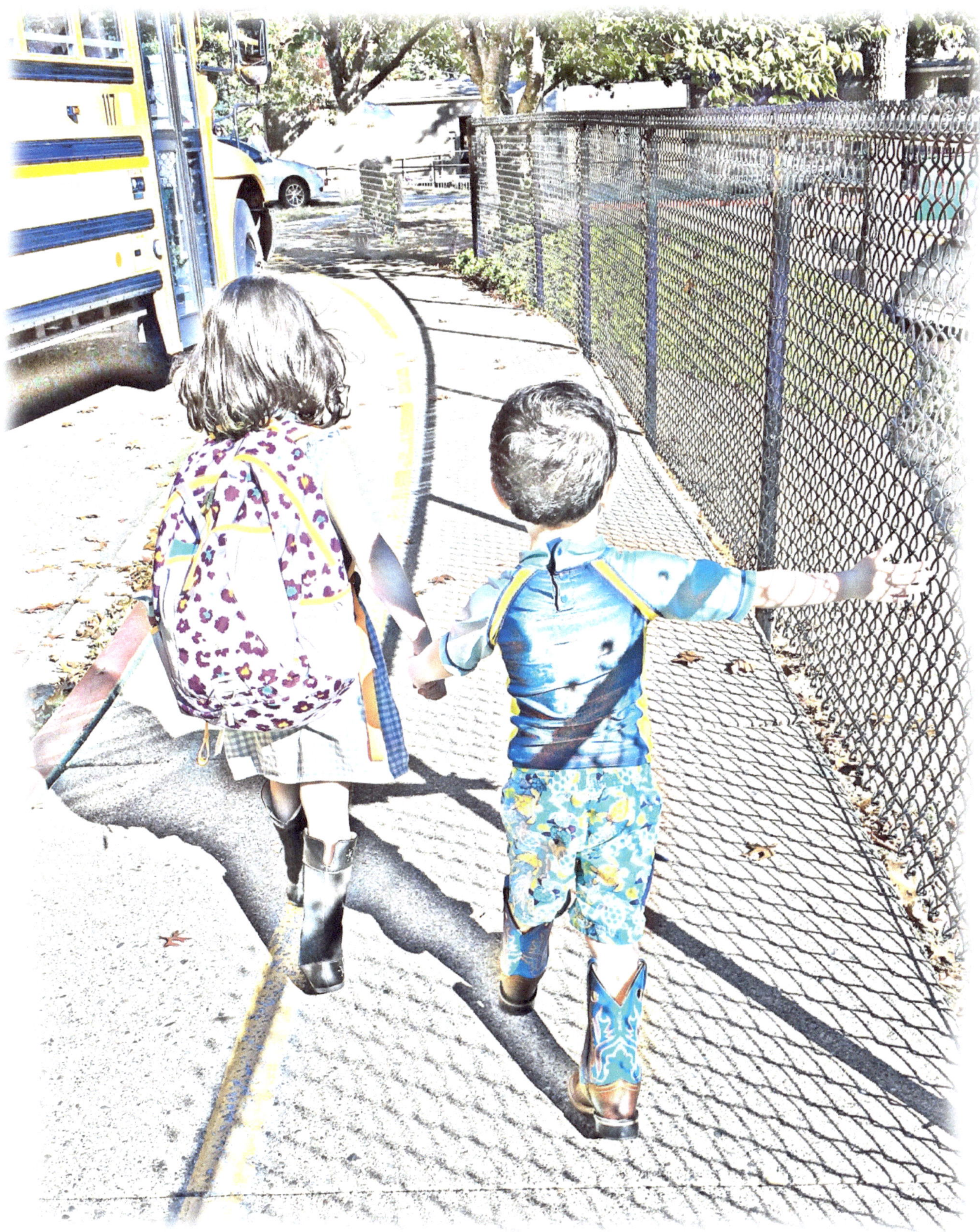

Mommy explained that there was something called a tumor in her chest. The tumor wasn't supposed to be there and it wanted to get bigger and make more tumors, like the weeds want to take over our garden. I hate weeding the garden, but I know that we have to pull out the weeds so that the vegetables can grow and be healthy.

Mommy told me that the cancer is kind of like weeds in her body. The cancer wants to spread and make it so her body can't be healthy just like the weeds want to spread and not let our vegetables be healthy.

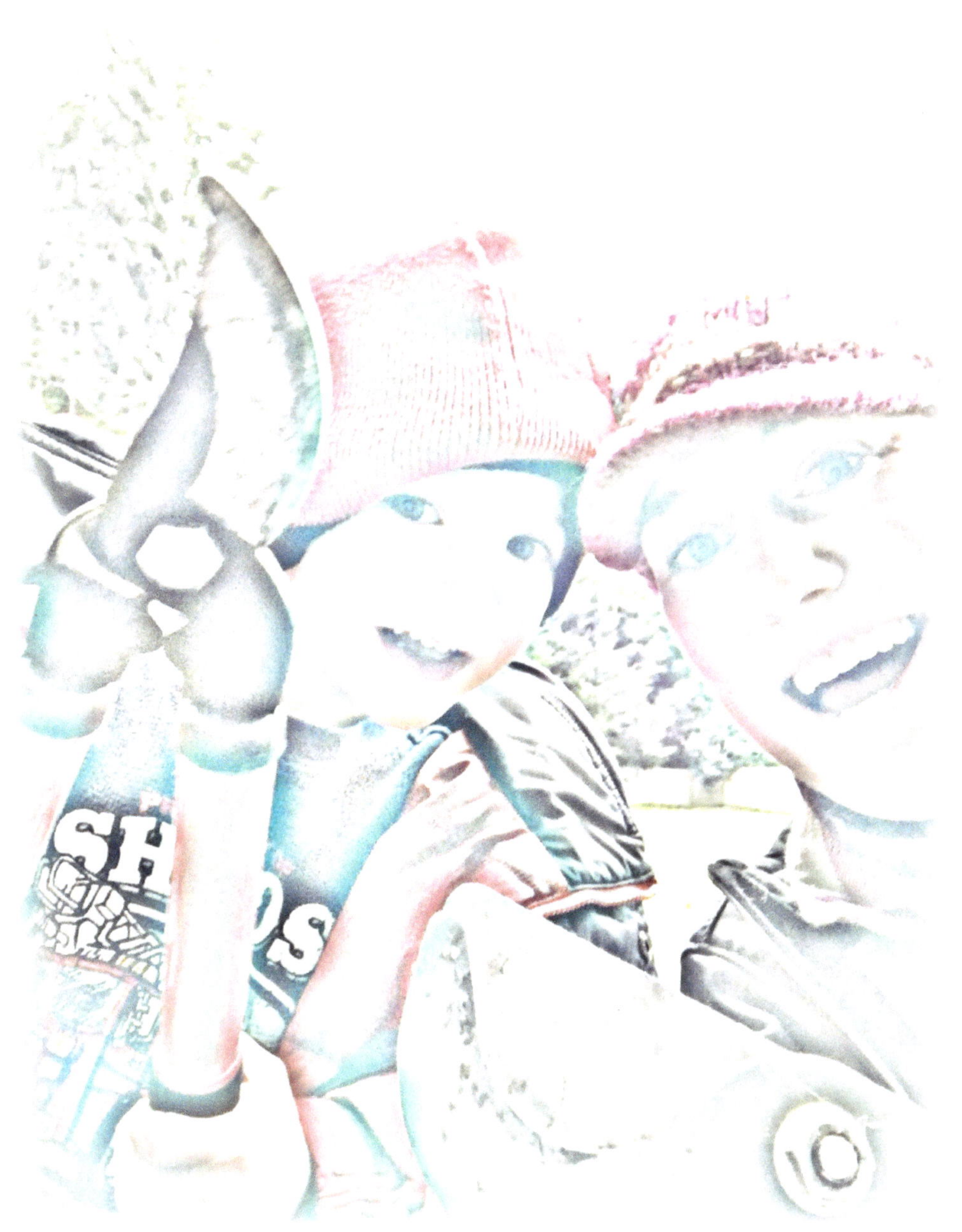

Mommy and Daddy let my little brother and me ask lots of questions. I asked Mommy if she was going to die. She told me she would do her very **very** best to fight the cancer because what she wanted most in the entire world was to be my mommy and my brother's mommy and to help us grow up. I wanted her to tell me she would be okay, but she said that with cancer it can be hard to tell for a while. I am glad she told me the truth, even though it wasn't exactly what I wanted to hear.

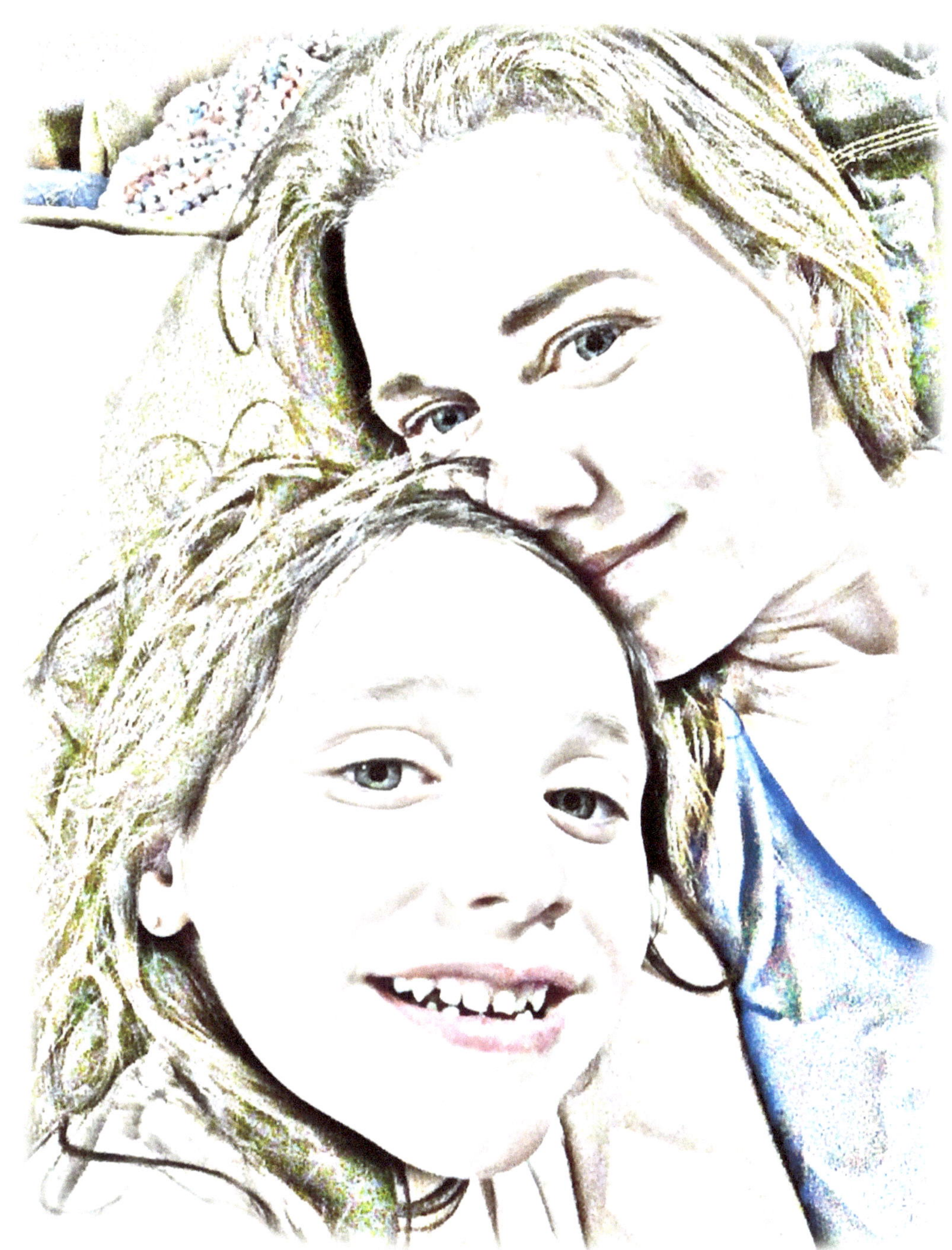

Mommy had lots of appointments with doctors. They did a ton of tests to figure out the best way to help Mommy to fight the cancer.

I got to meet Mommy's doctor and ask her lots of questions. She was really nice and super smart. I knew she would do her best to help Mommy get better.

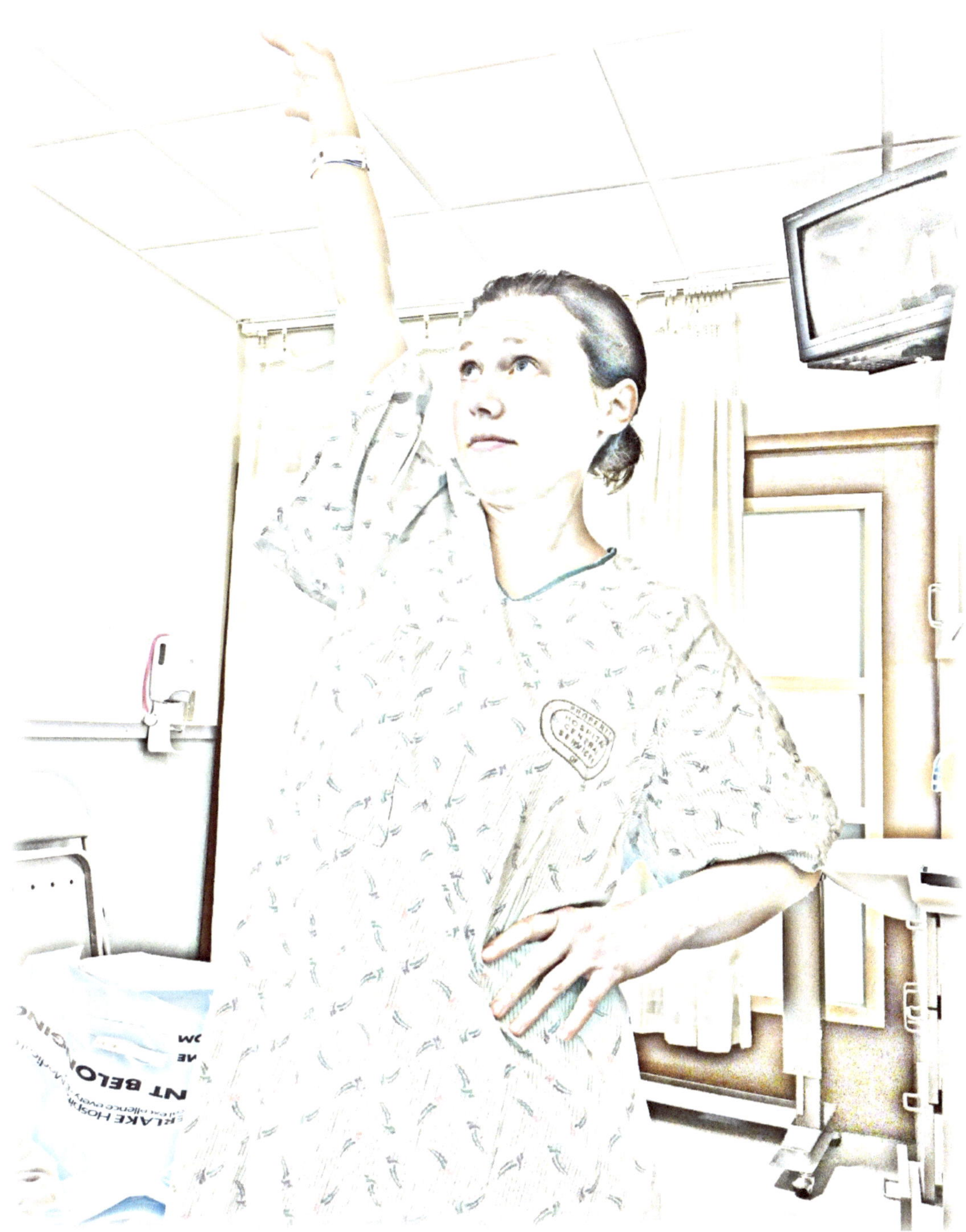

Mommy had surgery to get the caner out of her body. They called the surgery a double mastectomy. That means that the doctor removed both of Mommy's breasts. It made Mommy look different than what I was used to. I didn't mind that she looked different, I love Mommy no matter what she looks like.

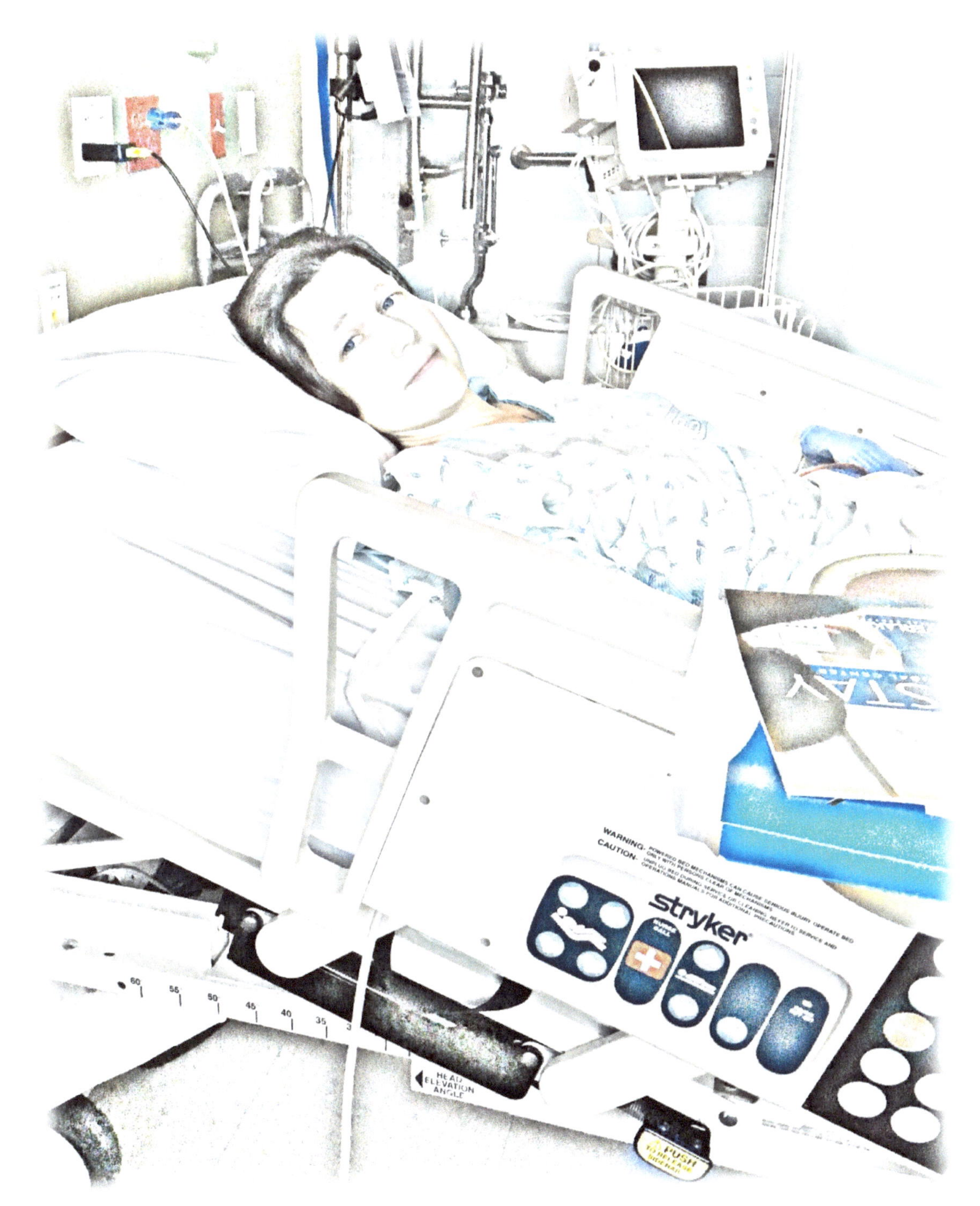
WARNING: POWERED BED MECHANISMS CAN CAUSE SERIOUS INJURY. OPERATE BED ONLY WITH PERSONNEL CLEAR OF MECHANISMS. REFER TO SERVICE BED
CAUTION: UNPLUG BED DURING SERVICE & OR CLEANING. SEE OPERATING MANUAL FOR ADDITIONAL PRECAUTIONS.
stryker
60 55 50 45 40 35
HEAD ELEVATION ANGLE
PUSH TO RELEASE SIDE RAIL

When Mommy got home from the hospital after the mastectomy, she hurt a lot. I had to be super gentle. My little brother and I couldn't give her big hugs or cuddle on her lap for a long time. She could barely give us hugs for weeks! That was so weird to not get hugs from Mommy, but she gave us lots of kisses.

I tried my best to help around the house because Mommy couldn't use her arms very much for a while. I set the table. I helped my daddy with the laundry. I even vacuumed the stairs! I was a great helper, and Mommy and Daddy really appreciated my hard work. My little brother tried to help too, but he didn't know how to do as much as I did.

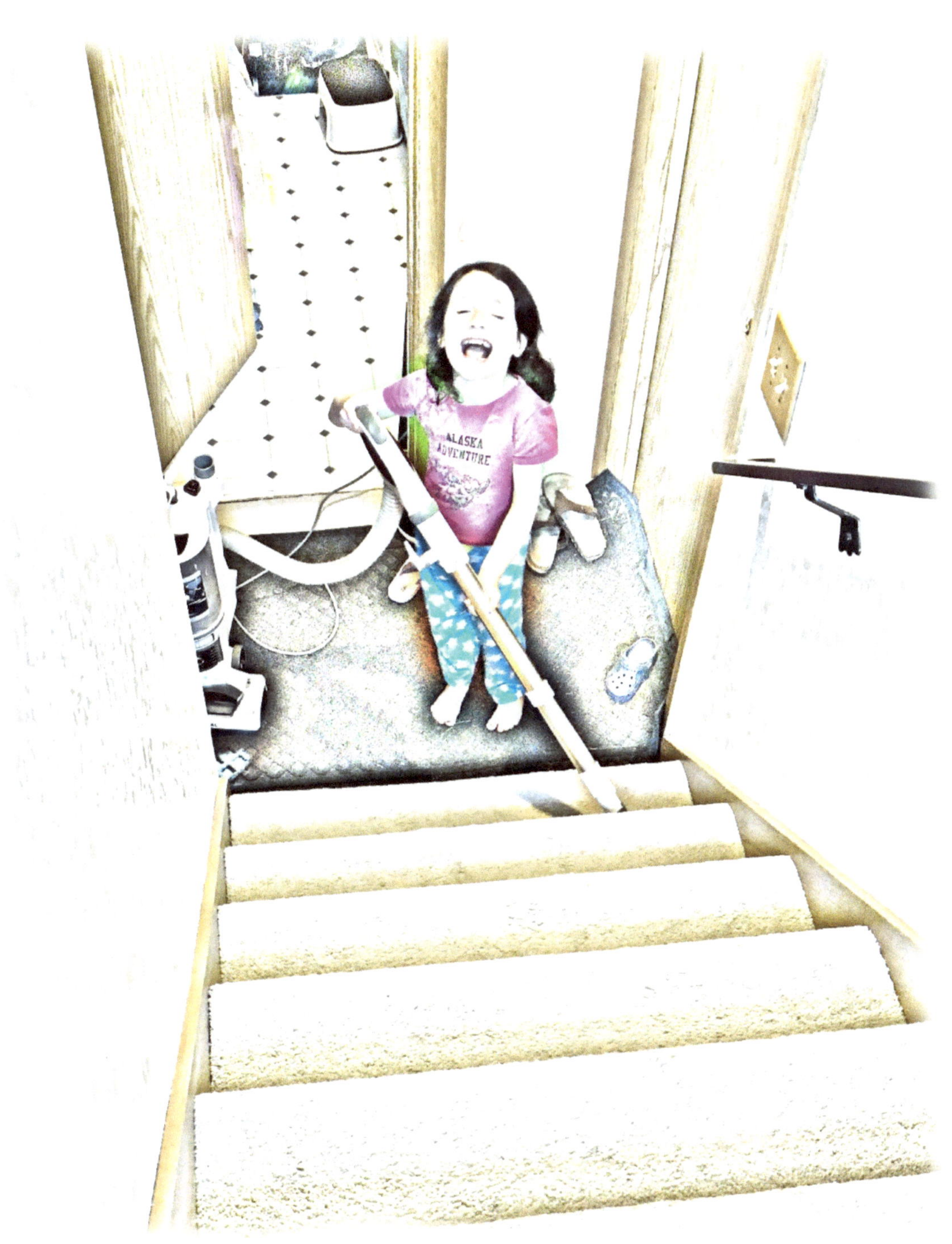

While Mommy started to recover from the mastectomy the doctor said that after taking a closer look at the cancer tumor that she thought Mommy needed medicine that they called Chemo. Mommy and Daddy explained that Chemo was really strong medicine that would make Mommy feel really sick. She would need to sleep a lot and she would have to be careful about a lot of things. She was even going to lose her hair! Mommy would have to have Chemo treatments for twenty weeks. That was a really long time.

Mommy decided that since she was going to lose her hair, that we should have some fun with it first. She let my little brother and me dye it any color we wanted. We chose pink since that is the color for breast cancer.

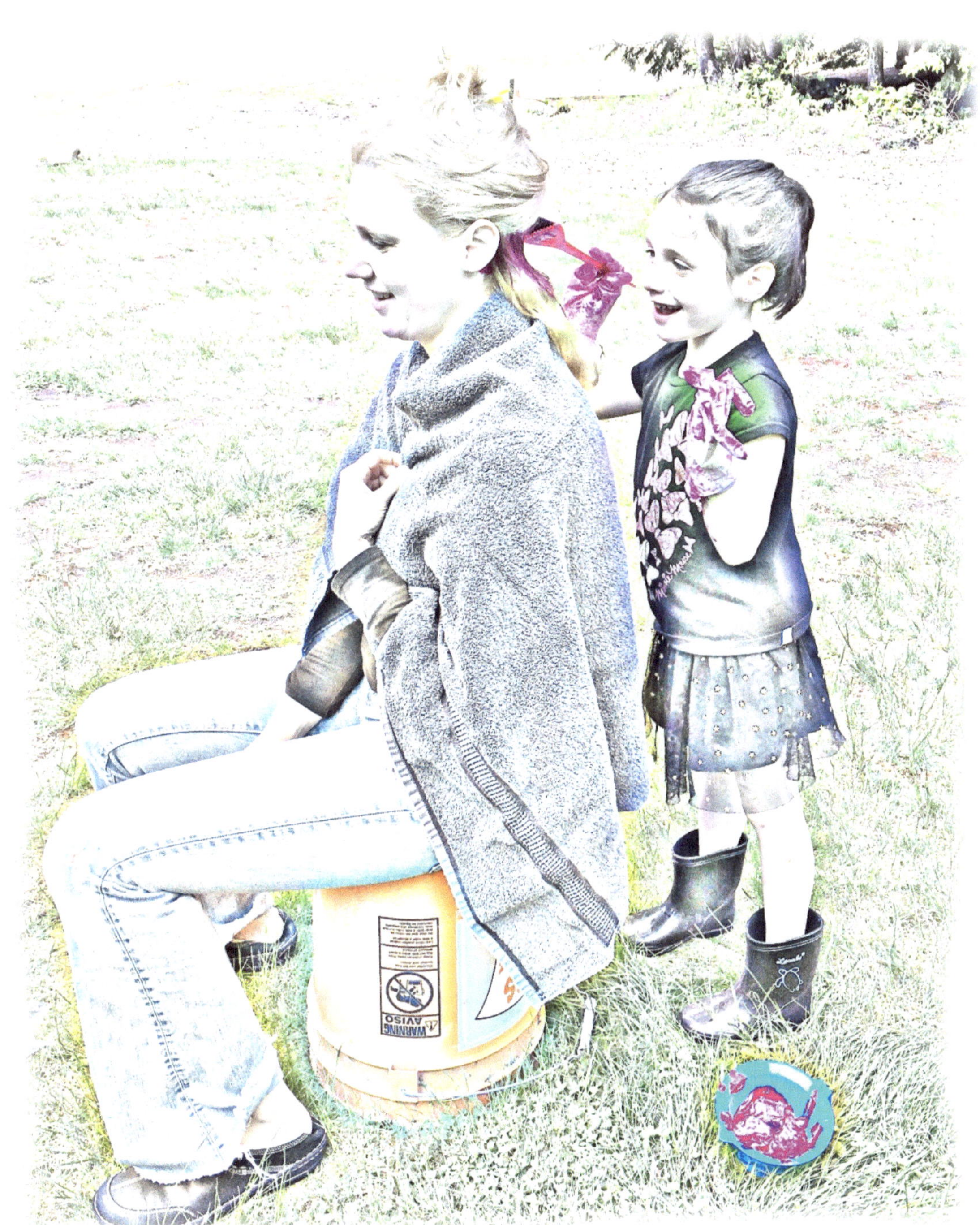

Mommy was going to need another surgery before the chemo started. The doctor needed to put a thing in Mommy's chest called a port. The port would help the strong Chemo medicine go into Mommy's body in a big blood vessel in her chest instead of a little one in her arm. Blood vessels are like tunnels all through our bodies for blood to flow through. Some are bigger than others. The biggest blood vessels are in our chests. Since the medicine that Mommy needed was super strong, the doctor wanted to put it in a big blood vessel so it would be able to mix with her blood quickly without hurting her.

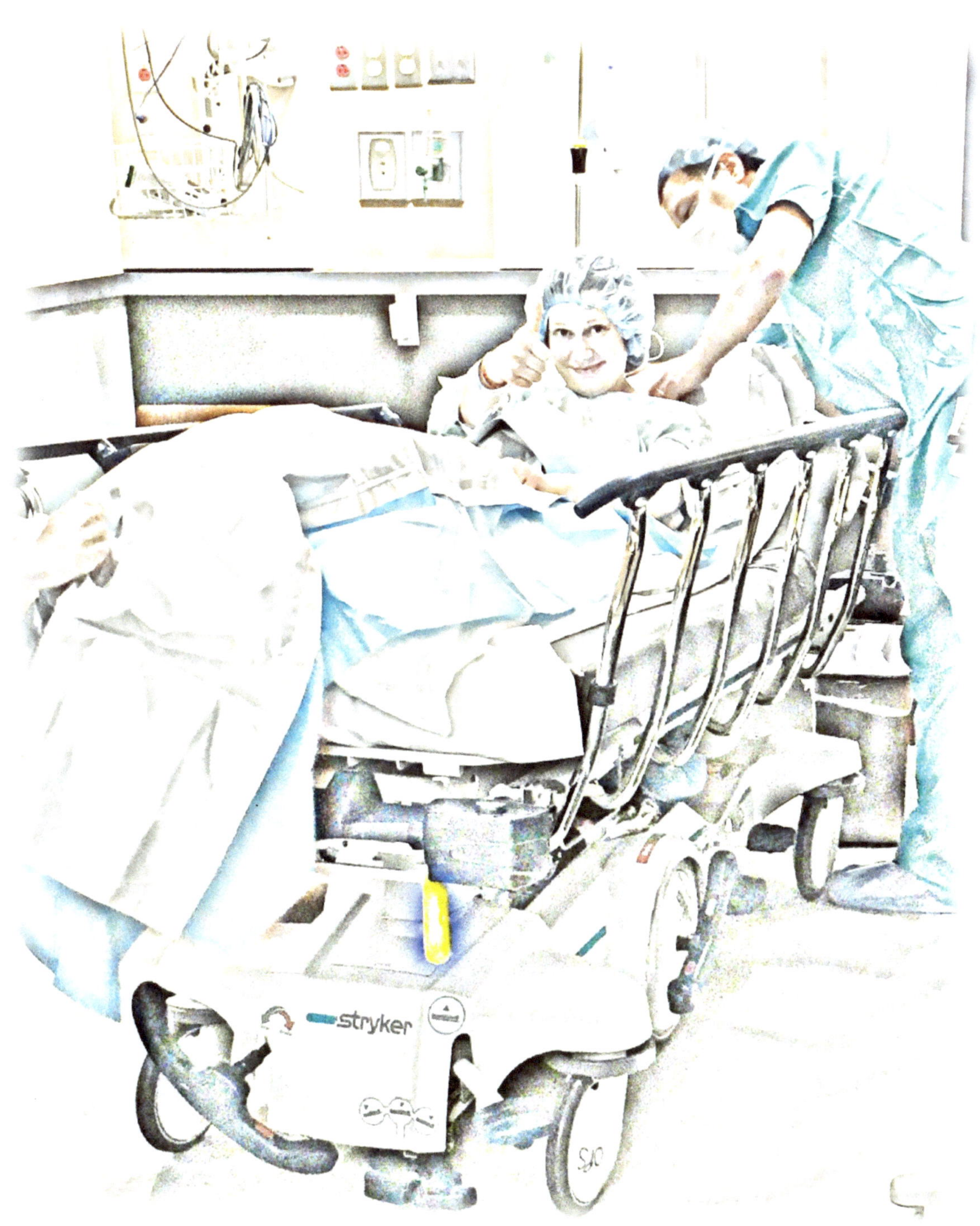
stryker

The surgery to put in the port was really fast. The port poked up from under Mommy's skin. It looked funny. I really wanted to touch it, but I had to wait until the bandages came off. When Mommy got the bandages off, she let me touch it. I had to wash my hands before and after I touched it and I had to be extra gentle. The port felt hard under her skin, harder than I thought it would. It was a little scary. I asked Mommy if it hurt. She said it did a little.

I was upset that Mommy was hurting. She told me that sometimes hurting isn't bad. She said that when we get an owie they sometimes hurt when they heal. She reminded me that sometimes I get growing pains when I grow, and I like getting taller. She also said that the things we work the hardest for we appreciate the most. She as working hard to get healthy, so she was going to appreciate her health when she got it back. I still didn't like that it hurt her, but I understood that the port was there to help her.

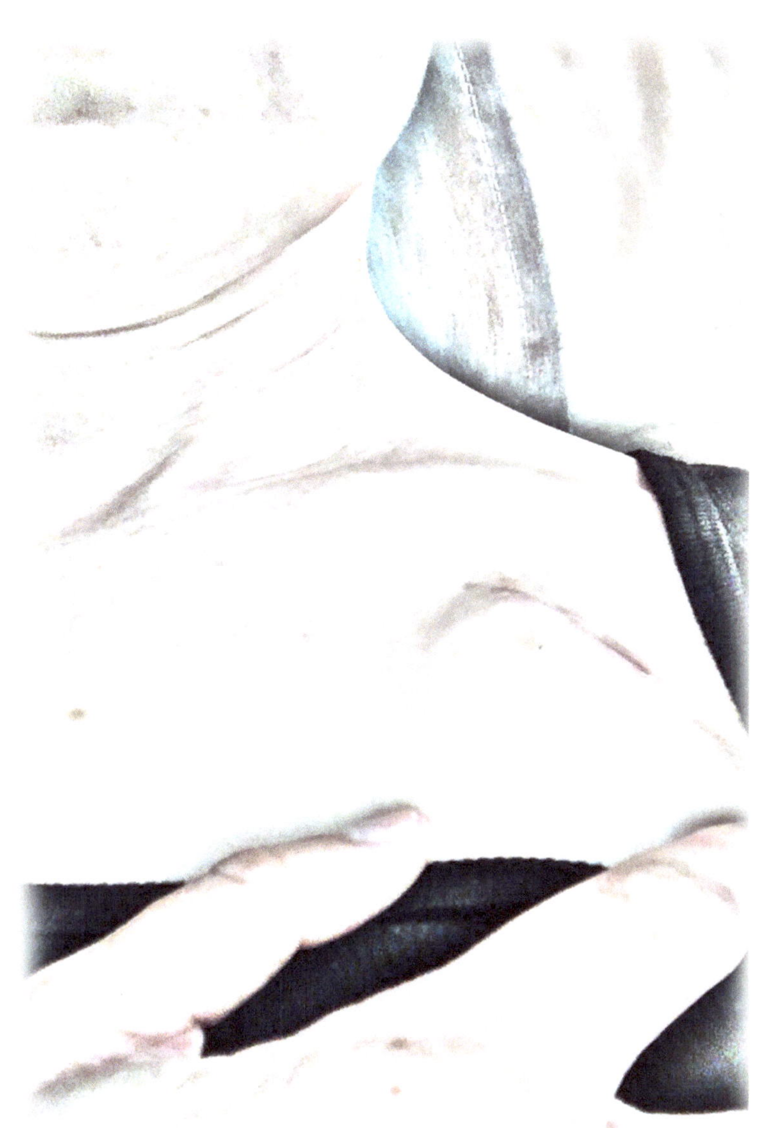

Daddy and my little brother went with Mommy to her first Chemo appointment, I had school that day. They both promised to take good care of her so I could go to school and not worry.

She needed to have a tube called an IV hooked up to her new port by a big needle. My brother said Mommy was really brave and the nurses were really nice. The nurses gave mommy medicine from big bags that hung up on a pole near Mommy and connected in to the IV and the port. The medicine was so strong that the nurses had to wear special paper clothes and rubber gloves that they took off and threw away after they set up the medicine and the IV. I'm not sure if that sounds more cool or scary. I guess a little of both. My little brother got to have some juice and snacks while he and Daddy waited for all the medicine from the bags to go into Mommy.

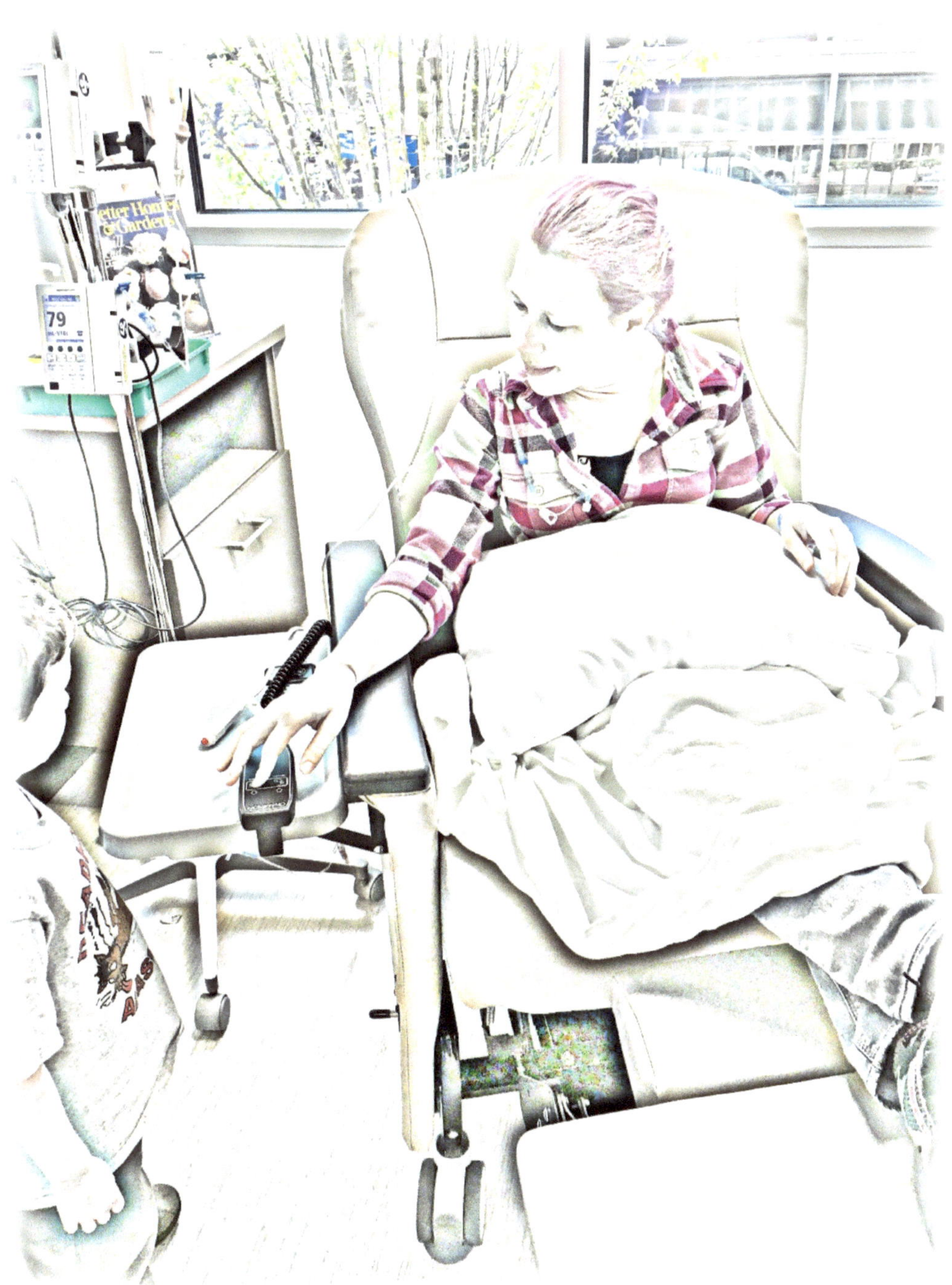

After mommy finished her medicine, they went home. They told me all about it when I got home from school. Mommy started to feel sick a little while later. Grandma came over to spend some time with Daddy, my brother, and me. Mommy had to go to bed pretty early. She felt really sick.

Mommy spent a lot of time in bed the next few days. Grandma and daddy took really great care of my brother and me and we all took great care of mommy. I liked to make sure that Mommy had plenty of water to drink. The doctor said it was really important for her to have lots and lots of water. I made sure to remind her to drink all her water and I kept plenty of water in her water bottle. Mommy said that the water I got for her tasted better than the water that anyone else got for her. I made the best water in the house. (The secret is just the right amount of ice.) Sometimes I would read to her, even though I had to make up some of the words.

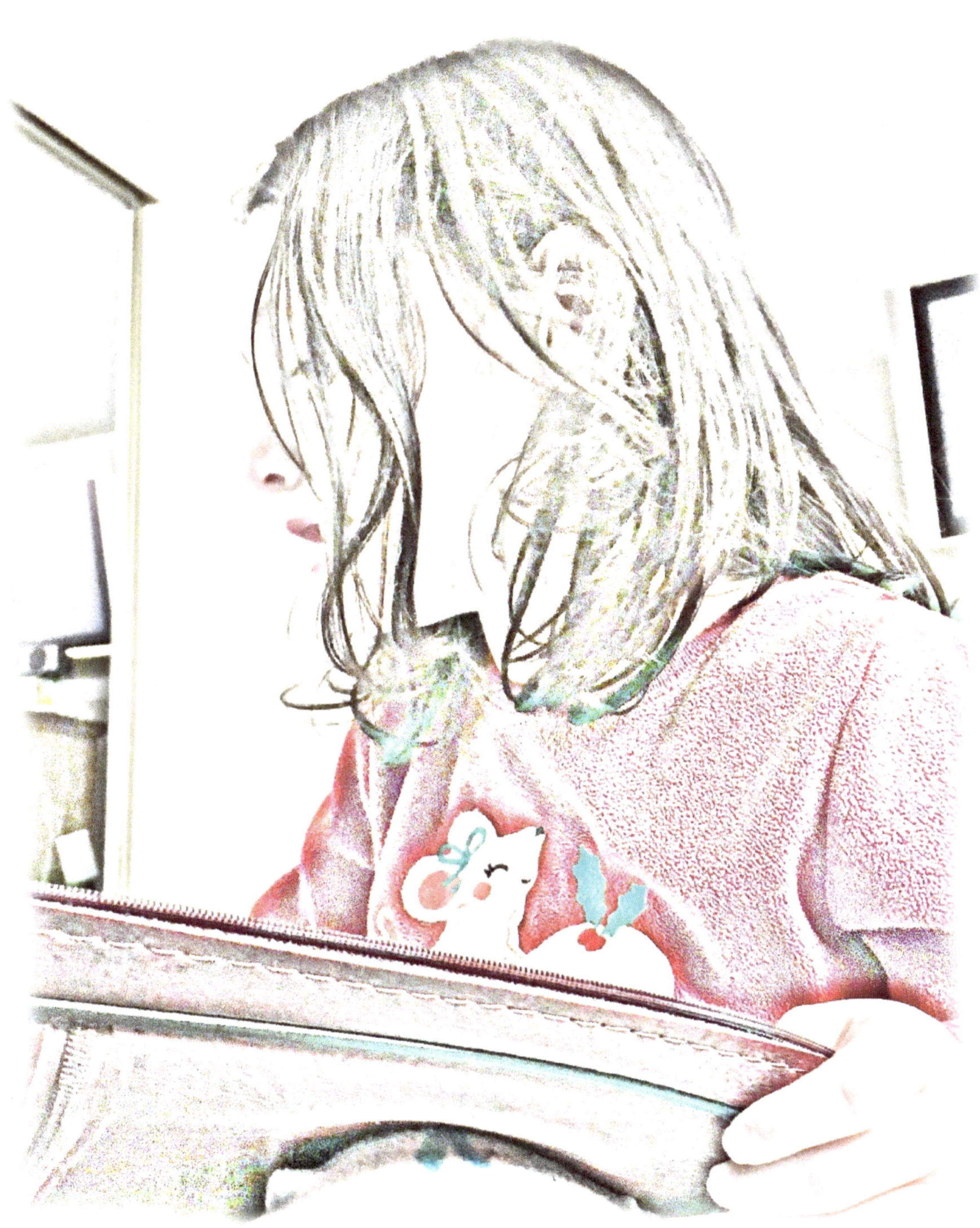

Mommy's hair started to fall out before the next Chemo appointment. As soon as it started to fall out, she decided it would be more fun to just shave it all off. I got to use the clippers to help shave Mommy's head! Daddy and I gave her a mohawk! It was awesome! We shaved the rest too, but only after we got some pictures of the mohawk.

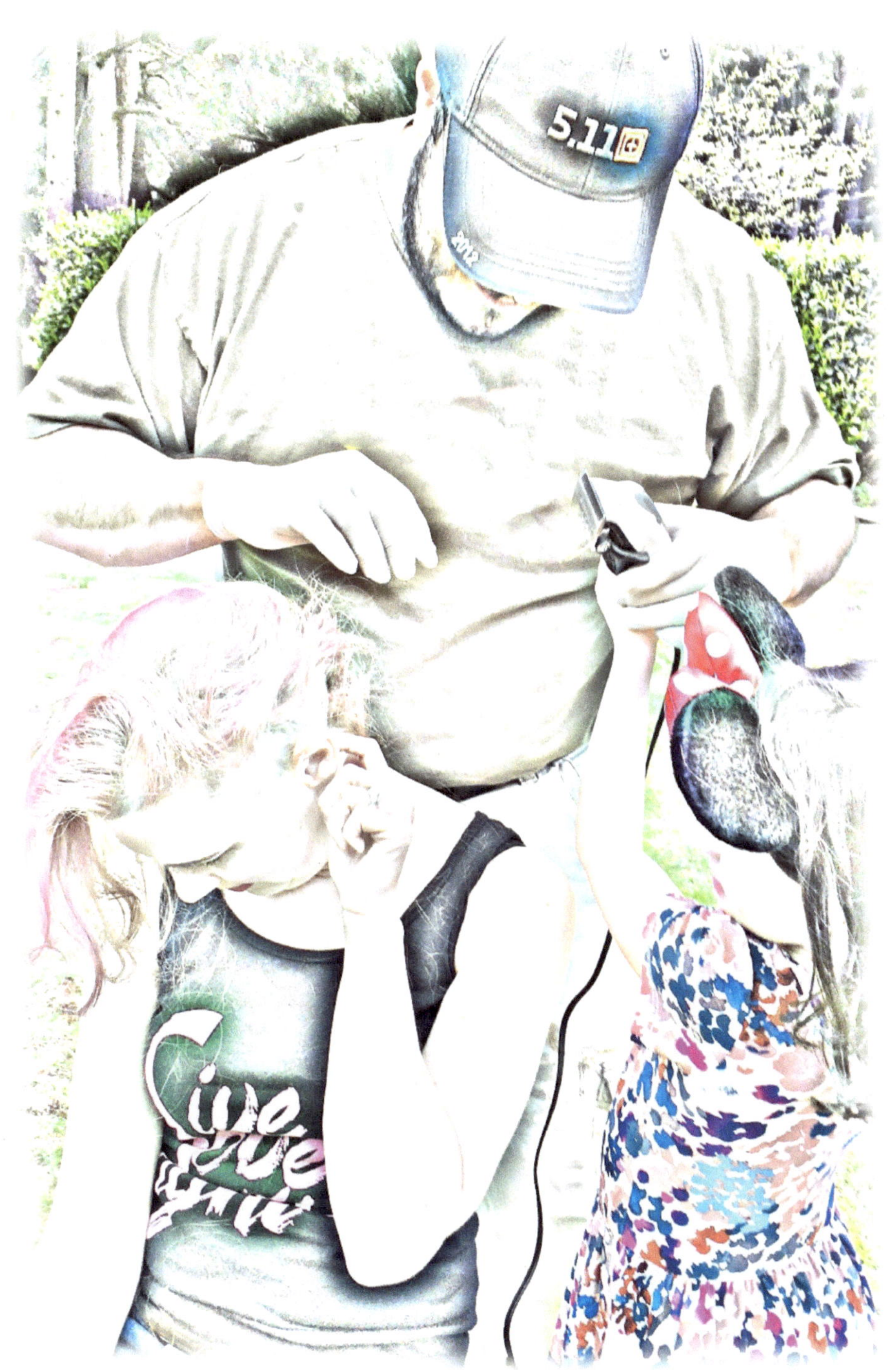

Some of my friends thought it was weird that my mommy didn't have hair. She explained to them that she had an infection called cancer and that she needed really strong medicine to get better, and that the medicine was so strong that it made her hair fall out, but it would grow back after she finished the medicine. Once she explained it to them, they seemed to understand.

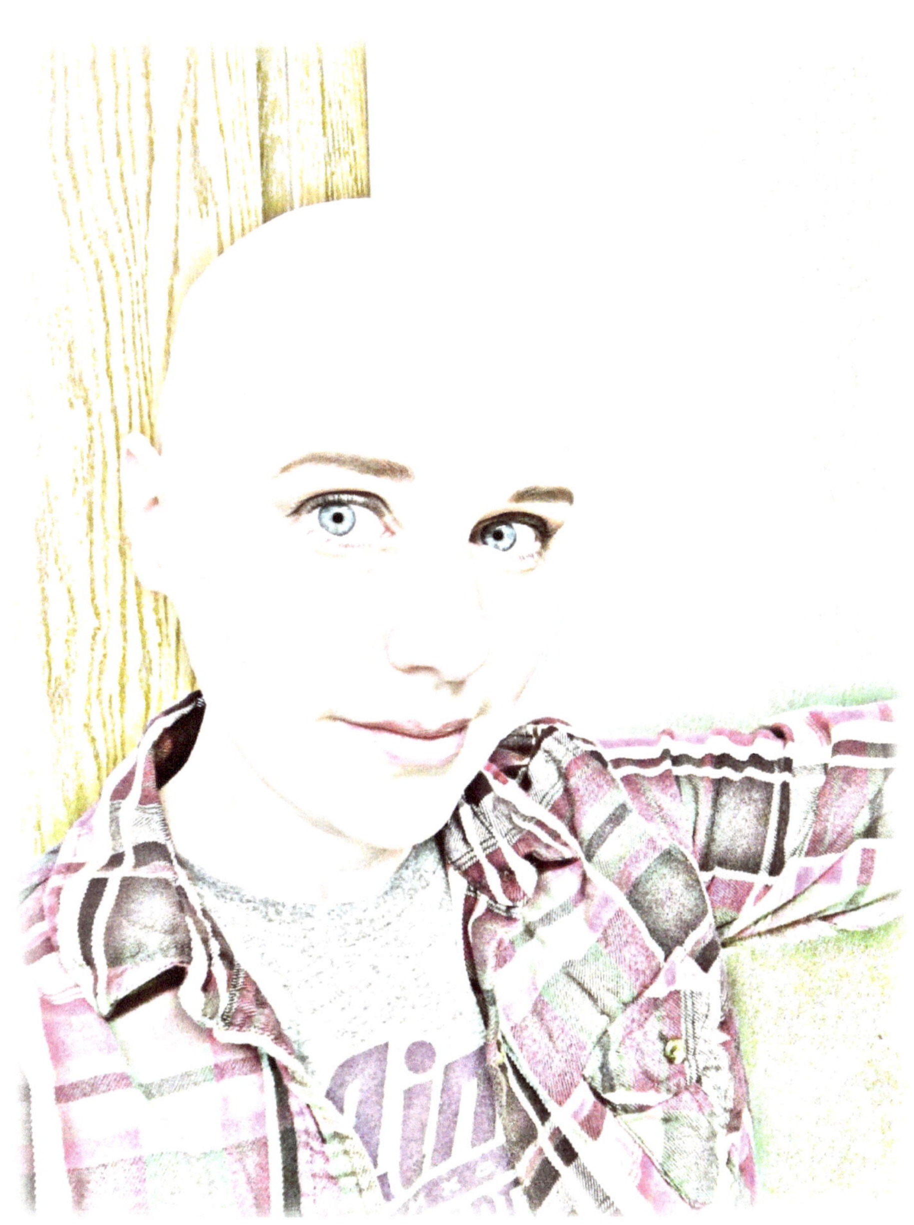

After Mommy had finished all her chemo treatments, she had to have another surgery to get the port taken out. She was excited to get the port out. I was happy to see Mommy excited.

Mommy said that sometimes people with breast cancer have to get more treatment called Radiation. Radiation is when doctors use special machines to send rays into where the cancer was to make sure they got it all. Mommy said that the rays can burn skin and make people feel sick, but it is worth it to try to get every bit of the cancer. Mommy didn't need radiation, but she told me she would have done it if the doctor recommended it. Some of the new friends she made during treatment got radiation. They said it was like a really bad sunburn. I've had sunburns before, they sting and can feel awful.

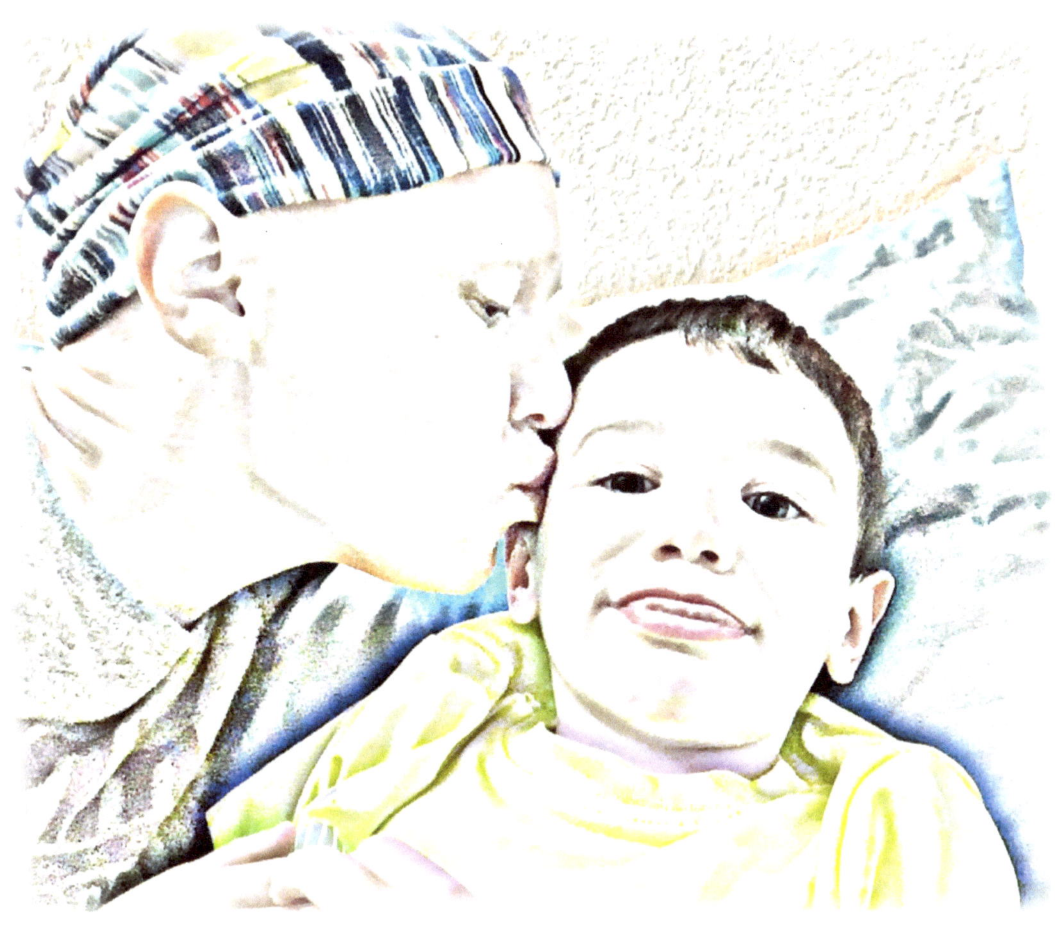

My mommy has a bunch of scars from the surgeries to get rid of her cancer. Some of them are pretty big, like the scars from the mastectomy surgery. I told Mommy that her scars are beautiful. They tell her story. They tell people how strong she is.

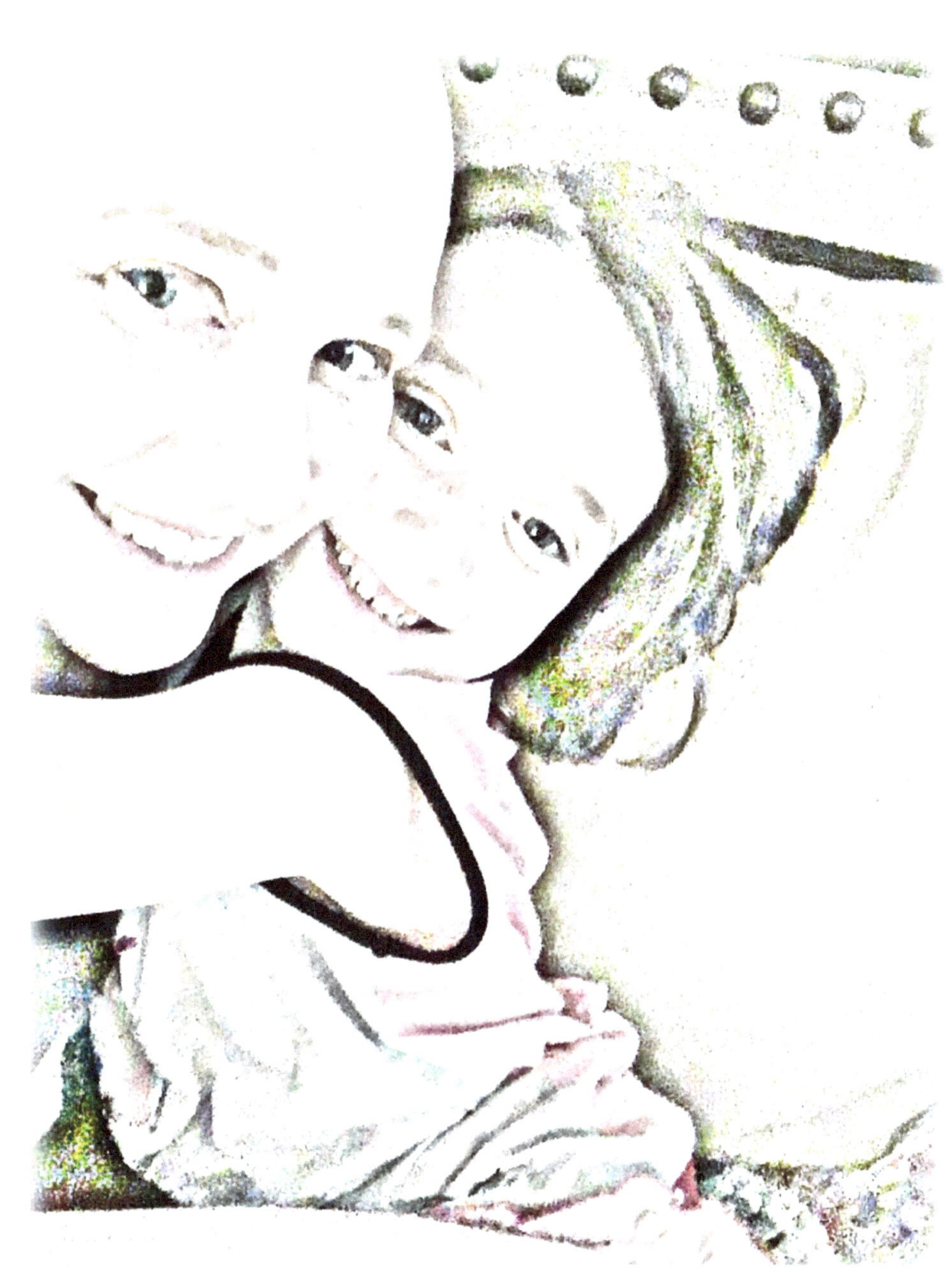

After mommy was all done with treatment, she decided to have reconstruction surgery. The doctor made new breasts for Mommy. Some of Mommy's friends chose not to get reconstruction. Mommy explained that each person who has a mastectomy has to choose for themselves if they want to have new breasts or not and that there are different ways doctors can build new breasts. There are different ways doctors can do this. Mommy got implants. They are kind of like water balloons under the muscle in her chest.

Soon, Mommy's hair started to come back. It was soft like a puppy. I liked to rub her soft puppy hair.

It took a while for Mommy to get strong again, but she didn't let that stop her from having fun with us!

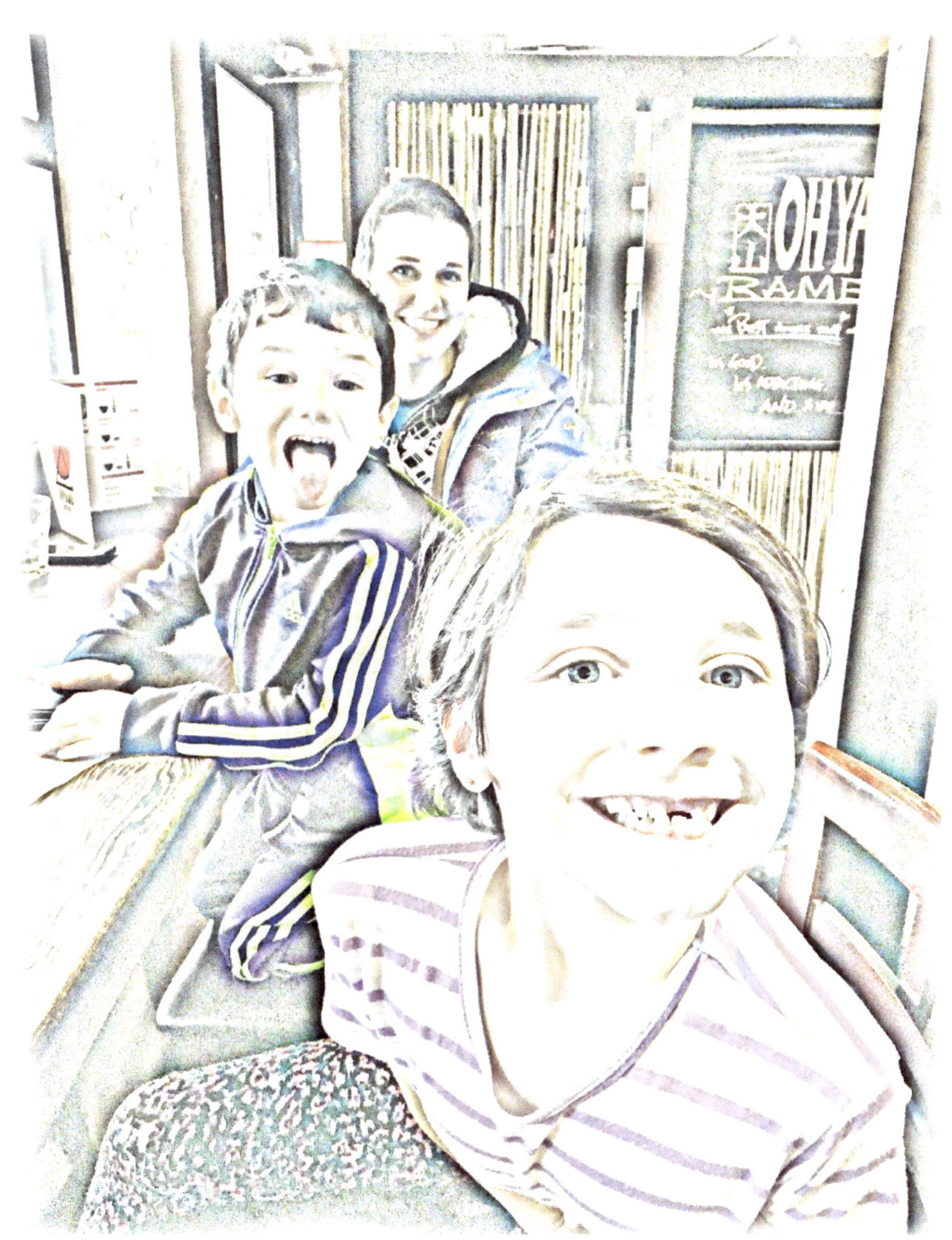

It's been **two years** since Mommy finished all her treatment and she is doing great! We are all thankful for every day we get with Mommy, and she is thankful for every day she gets with us.

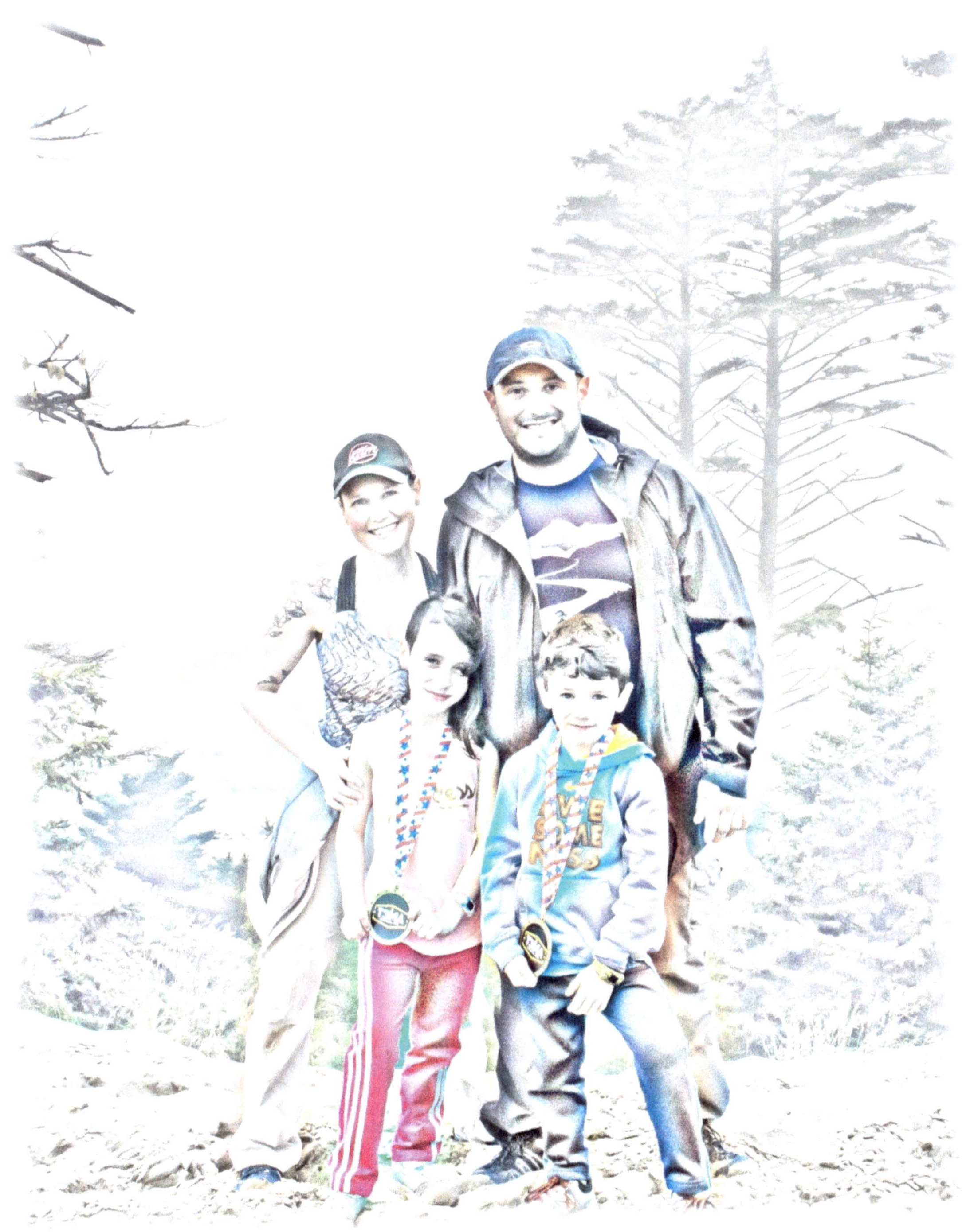